THE SECRET TO DIET

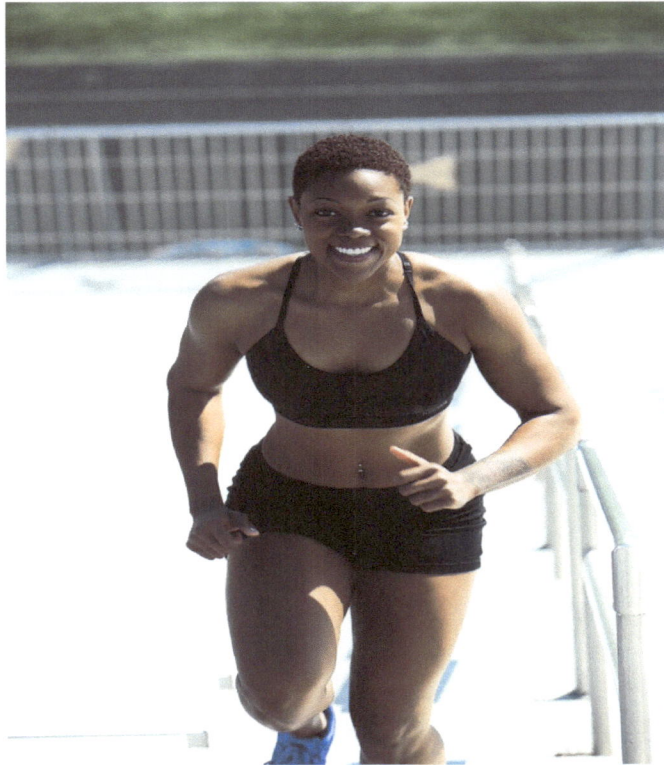

By JJ Schousboe

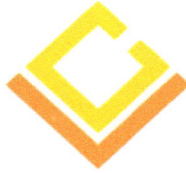

JJ LEARNING CURVE, LLC
To An Amplified Life- Bridging the gap from
academics to your life's achievement

The Secret to Diet
By JJ Schousboe

Copyright (c) 2018 JJ Learning Curve, LLC
First Edition – December 2018

ISBN: 978-0-359-31935-0

Produced by
Lulu Press, Inc.
627 Davis Drive
Suit 300
Morrisville, NC 27560

Table of Contents

Introduction

I wrote this book to help you gain insight and to open up your thoughts, about the different aspects of diet, dieting and maintaining it. In the six areas of life, health and balance is on of which may need support for change and growth. Everyone at some time has changed their diet, or worked on it. Here you will get added information to help you to make some different choices, which are your own and will work for you.

You may or may not have looked at some of these areas before now. In this book, you can dive further to learn what will work best for you, to not only achieve weight loss but to keep it off. This information walks you through ten areas for clarity about what it takes and how you can get there.

You can always remember that everything which we may do takes some time and therefore we learn in the process of going through the actions. I have added my personal healthy foods and recipe tips, for your new experience and enjoyment.

Start to practice what works for you, by making it your new habit. It is that simple after reading this book and attaining, "The Secret to Diet."

To Your Health!

JJ Schousboe

Acknowledgment

Thanks to my business partner for being my first case study and sharing with me her personal challenge, which aided me in discoveries to share with you in this book.

Some Signs of Being Over Weight

Check List

Even though your mind may be comfortable with your weight, or the way that you look, here are some points to consider and do your self check to see if you need to follow some of the advice given in this book. Also to have a better understanding for your, "Why" you may need to do this as you learn how.

Remember that your health can, or should be your first cause.

- You may get tired and/or breathless more frequently.
-
- Your feet and back may hurt.
-
- Your legs rub together when you are not wearing pants.
-
- You are no longer comfortable wearing high heels shoes.
-
- You get the cold and flu more frequently.
-
- You have a great appetite.
-
- Your weight is higher than the average height to age ratio.

One

Its Not About Food

In today's information world (whether on line or in books), there are a wide variety of topics on diet, exercise, nutrition and health. You can see this also on the news and by media advertisements. The topics all lends to give advice on the latest trends and discoveries, as the information become available to the public.

You are now here to discover that there is a missing piece of the news puzzle. An essential part to diet. It may not be what you have been told, or what you maybe thinking. The secret will be out to you.

You may or may not have heard about this secret but even if you have, it was not told to you, in this way. You now have a link to begin applying it with your diet plan, to achieve your goal.

WHAT IS DIET

Diet is the amount of food consumed by a person. It implies the intake of food for nutritional values. What ever you eat (which can range by cultural differences) is your diet.

Your food intake may or may not give you the correct amount of nutrients, which you need daily. However, it is your food choice or daily-eating habits.

We all need meat for protein. Beans are second for protein but cannot replace it. Vegetables and fruits for vitamins, potassium, fiber, iron, calcium, magnesium and so on. We need carbohydrates to provide energy to our bodies. Some are sugar, glucose, fructose sucrose and lactose. These are what fuel our muscles to maintain our physical activities.

Although many people today choose to become vegetarians, maintaining health and weight, still needs to have a balance intake of nutrients. With all the food choices we have already discussed, planning a menu can easily be done, based on your needs for nutritional intake.

The bottom line is when you are planning to stick to a daily diet (intake of food), it is important to consider, there long term nutritional value, (for optimal health benefits), and easy daily maintenance of the diet.

Food is a source of not only nourishment, which we need to survive, it is a form of socializing and enjoyment. In today's standard of productivity, especially (here) in the United States, we have a wide array of food choices, from all the nation's cultures.

We have restaurants offering all that you can eat, for breakfast, lunch and dinner. Our supper markets are specializing in organic products for healthy living choices, as our information on new research for health are discovered.

It is now quite easy to make a menu to eat healthy, by ordering planned meals, which can be delivered to your door. They include recipes with measured ingredients, ready to assemble and cook, in little time.

However, if you find that they are too expensive, you can hop over to the local fruit and vegetable location and easily make a chicken salad from scratch. This maybe a simply, healthy choice to consider as a meal. I can go on further about our food choices and our nutrition knowledge, but by now you got the point. They are readily available to us almost everywhere.

Therefore, when we look at diet in the develop world, **the right kind of food is not the problem**, or even access to it. We have the choices. So what is keeping us from achieving our diet goals?

It not about food. Lets read on to find out.

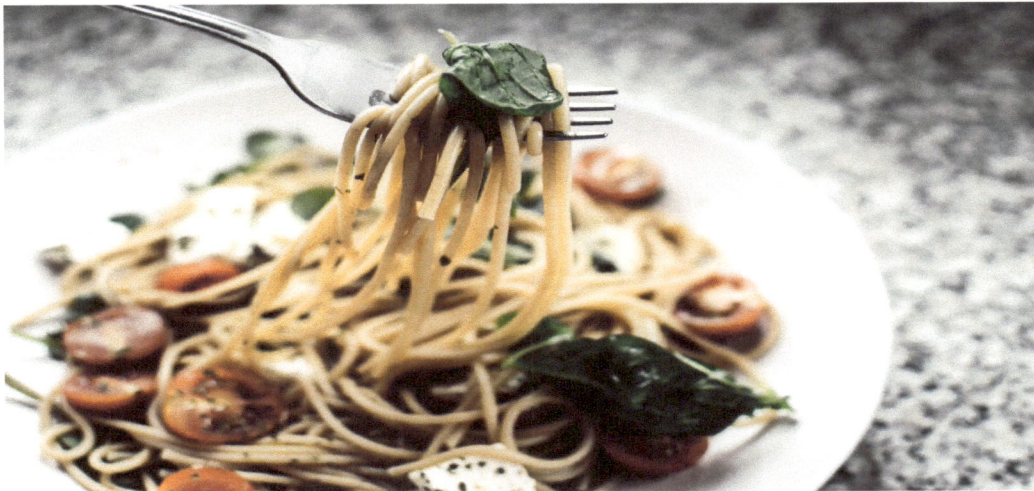

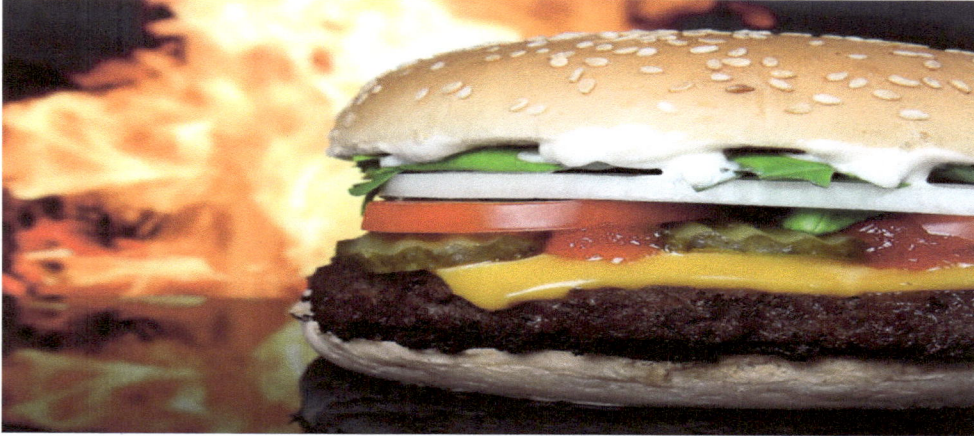

Finding the Right kind of Food is Not the Problem

Two

Its NOT Fasting

Fasting, is one form of diet some people adopt. Some may believe, that if you don't eat a lot of food, you can not gain weight. Indeed fasting is hard to maintain, hardly ever works and can lead to disorders. Here is why.

Of all the food choices which are available to us, we are not just choosing, to eat or not. We live in a time of advertisements. We are surrounded by them. We are being enticed to shop and eat. Although we need to be responsible, we must recognize external input in what we do.

We are also learning, that even colors in the restaurants are chosen and geared to entice our appetites and cause us to eat. So, even thought some people may take the fasting route, they can still become enticed and loured, by food advertisements and displays.

Personally, I have found myself wanting my food order from a restaurant, to look exactly like the picture, on the beautiful laminated menus, which I receive to order from. The kicker is, (for some) after eating by enticement, the guilt comes in, and fasting seems like the next best way, of getting rid of over eating.

In many cases society can challenge us in believing that we will be more liked, if we are skinny. Although, some of us think that having some weight can help us not to be bullied, or be pushed around. We cannot decide what we are comfortable with, so gaining and losing weight, becomes a yo yo, pattern of behavior.

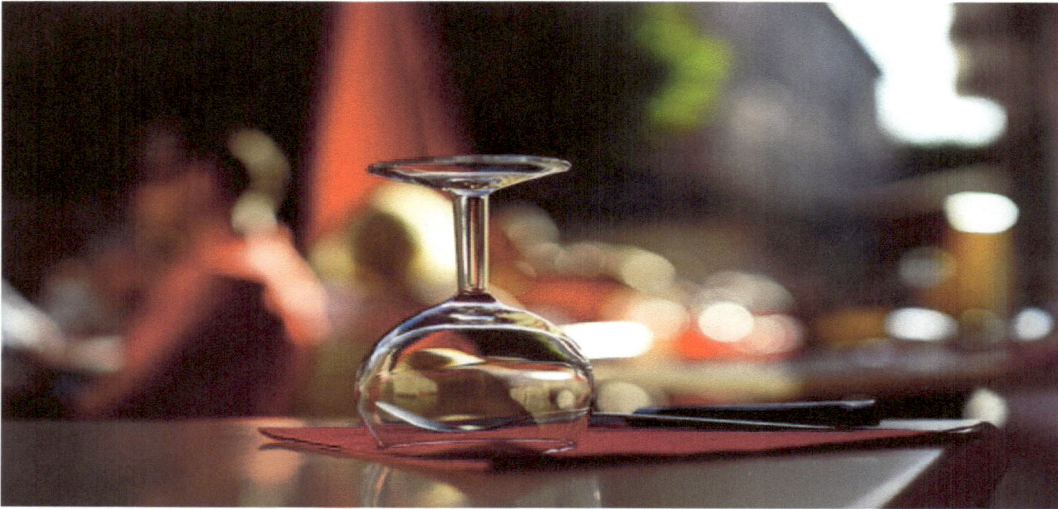

This pattern has a name. It is called an "Eating Disorder." It can get even more in depth by inducing, vomiting and purging. The human mind is very adaptable to patterns and habits. When anything is repeated a couple of times, the mind forms an acceptable pattern and makes it a habit, almost as a law to live by.

Don't get me wrong here. If you fast for a day for religious or cleansing purposes, it is a clear choice, and that choice is not based on managing diet, or weight gain.

Fasting based on guilt of over eating and food consumption, is what can form a destructive habit. It can then take a life time to cure. When this occurs, help will definitely be needed to overcome the disorder, or habit.

Another point is, skipping breakfast alone, can trigger the primal fear of hunger response to eat more. This can also cause your appetite to be over stimulated. And, in turn, it can effect your digestive system, cause gas, blotting and constipation, including weight gain. If you get to the point of malnutrition long tern, it can also affect your body's immune system. On those previous points, fasting is not recommended for diet.

About Maintaining Diet, it is Not Fasting

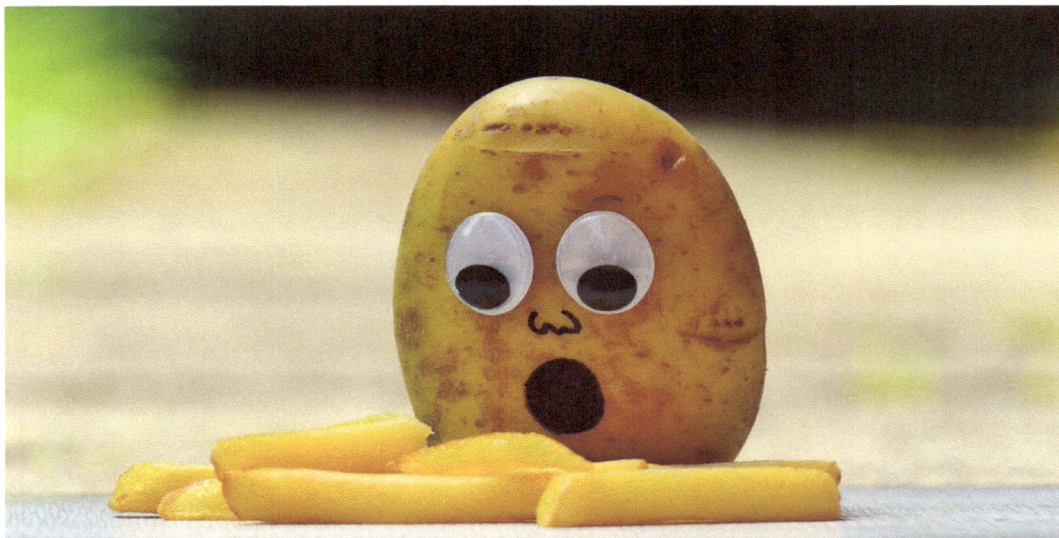

No food? Well its not about fasting.

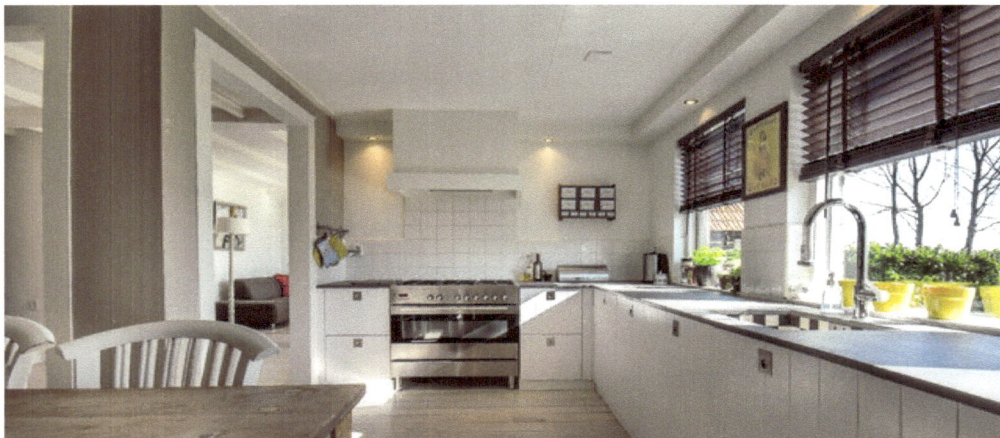

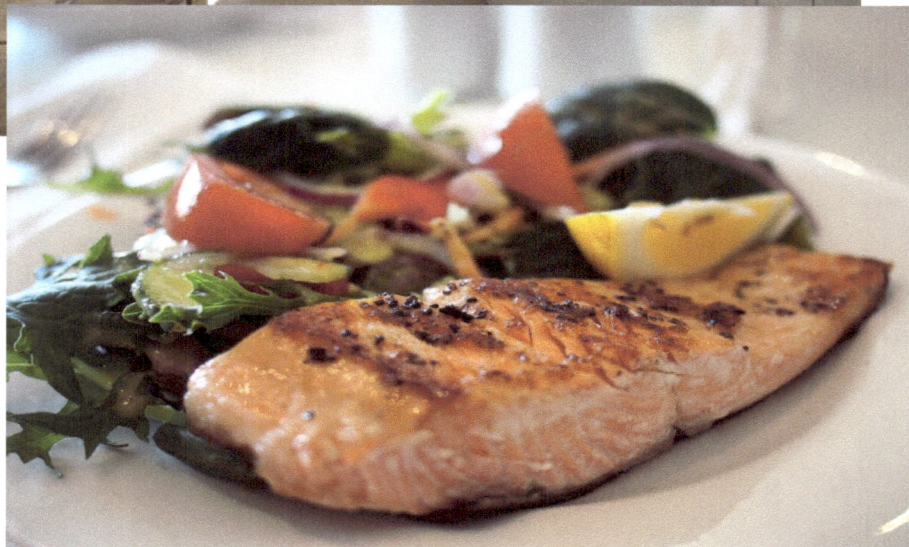

Three

It is Not the Right Plan for You

Have you ever tried to diet and found yourself going from one plan to another? After many attempted plans, you find out that they simply does not work for you? Many others have done it, (you think) so why can't I do it?

You experience year after year, of dieting and loosing weight, then regaining it as soon as you stopped. Yes? Is this you? Are you nodding your head to this question right now? I have known people, who has done this personally. I have heard their stories.

Now you can get the answer here. I can tell you that it is not the plan, as a life and relationships coach. The plan that is right for you is yet to be discovered in this book.

Here is why it is not about you finding , "The Right Plan."

There are several diet plans and dietary experts out there. They all have their plan and claims that it works. So, how can you know which one is the right one for you? Until you have tried several of them, you may not be able to decide which one work and can be the right one for you. It is like going to the doctor to find the right treatment for your symptoms and not finding the cause.

If you look at diet plan like medicine, you may not be able to tolerate the side effects of some medicine. You may unknowingly be allergic to a drug and have to stop it and try another or different kind. When you choose a plan before accessing information on the it, you can go through that trial and failure process.

Some diet plans contain high fats, which are supposed to be the good kinds of fat for our body. High fat however, can cause break outs or pimples, if you already have oily to medium skin types. If you break out after these kinds of diet stop and change them at once.

Other types of diets offers little fibers. Fibers are needed for regularity. If you are on a liquid diet, you may need to add salad or a green drink for fibers intake, to maintain balance.

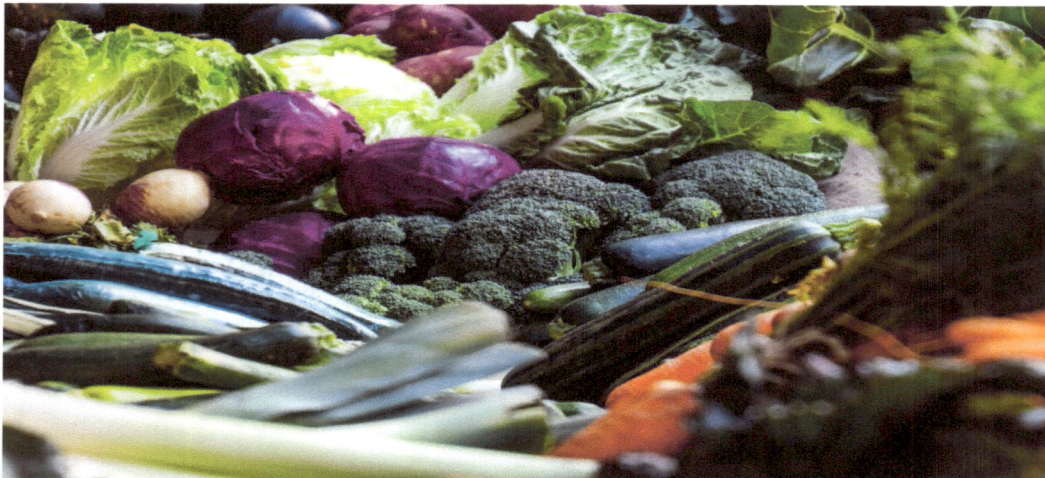

Somehow once again, after you feel that you have the right plan, you cannot stop it, or you regain the weight, which you had before you began.

You did everything as your plan instructed you to. It works for you it seems. Here the kicker is however, that what works for you, you are now on it, for the rest of your life.

It becomes like taking a prescription drug for a medical condition. This was not what you had in mind, when you got started on your diet plan, I am sure.

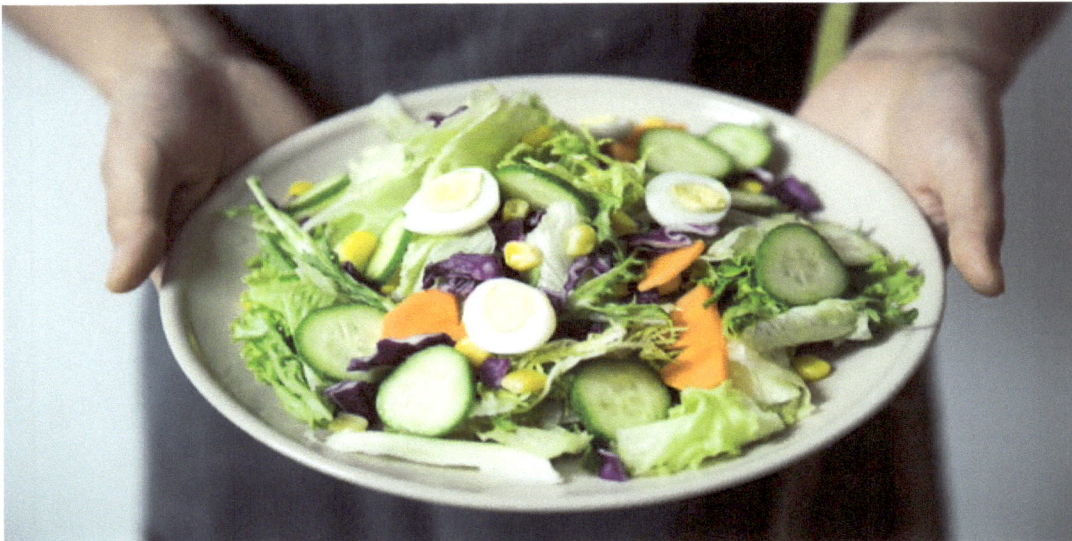

Its not the perfect diet plan for me.

What we have previously discussed are some of the reasons why so many people start a diet and stop, or give up on dieting all together. Some people have found that it simply does not work for them, the way that they had imagined it would. Living by choice and freedom, is not what they feel when they think about diet and having to maintain a plan for life.

So let us move on to a more positive approach, and share with you insight that can aid you in, **"the secret" of what can really work for you.**

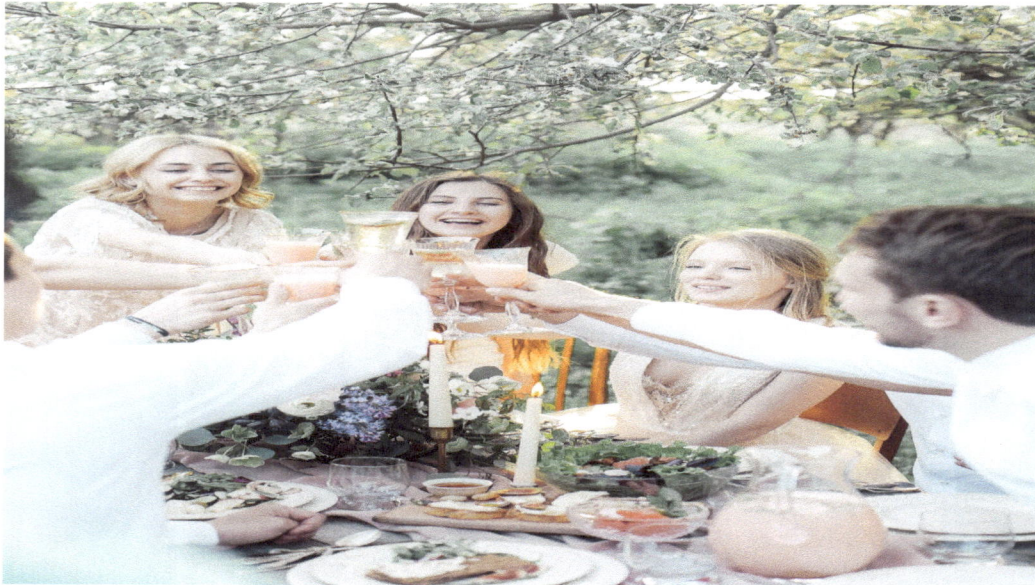

Four

The Purpose of Weight

An aspect to consider is the purpose of weight gain. Why do we gain weight, is not only because of food or fat intake but also with our increased age. Have you ever considered that? Why is this so?

It is a natural part of our age in growth. This is a stage that is not taught or accepted, as a factor why we are no longer a size 8 or 10, but a 12 or 14 in our clothing. A woman can be unhealthy to conceive at age 30, if she is 100 pounds, whether she is 4 or 5 feet in height. Weight increase has its benefits, as we age. Let's look into that further.

We look at growth, as we stop growing up wards, as an adult. We are taught that we stop growing around 18 to 21 years of age. We are not taught that we are still growing. In fact we are growing, but outwards. We gain more mass to support more activity. Our body can then support our age appropriate lifestyle. For example, motherhood and fatherhood.

In our aging process we will naturally eat less food and consumed less sweets. The weight at an older age, may not be as needed to give way to our lifestyle support, compared to when we are younger, and more active.

The aging process also gives less regeneration which takes up more energy and nutrients to give performance, for the youth functions of the body.

In other words weight gain and weight loss is a natural part of aging. It is part of the cycle of life. We go from growing upwards to growing outwards. Hips speed to sit longer, as our feet give way to tiredness or poor health. We become lighter with age as well, so that we can be easily assessed to be cared for.

We can look at it as, caring for a baby and an older person, is easier to manage. My mother use to say, "Once a man, twice a child." That saying works both for our mental and physical progression, or regression, in our aging process.

I have heard that weight gain is blamed on some preservatives in our food supply. This may be so, but it is not the only factor to consider. Understanding that weight gain is a natural process takes the frenzy away, from control, to management. We may need to work on being healthy and comfortable, in our movement and mobility, no matter what age group we are currently living in.

Exercise to Stay fit, Energized and Build Mussels

We all know and understand the value of exercise. Exercise works not only for keeping off, or maintain weigh gain, but also to keep us mobile and give us energy. Exercise can also build our mussels to give us strength, to support a healthy lifestyle. Exercising is the outer source of our weight control plan. However, exercise can cause you to become more hungry when starting a diet plan. Let us look at the many ways in which to exercise.

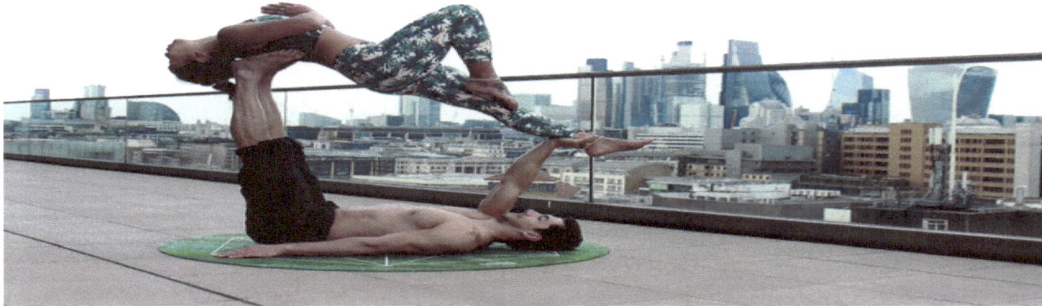

Exercising for strength and health.

Choosing which form of exercise is best for you will depend on may factors. You must consider your health condition, along with your age and weight. It is also advised to consult with a physician before choosing a vigorous or most form of exercise.

There are many instructors who will work with you either one on one, or within a group. Yoga is a form of group exercise that is calming and slow, but will work the whole body for you. Check if this will suit your goal needs and enjoy the group support as well.

Maintaining weight needs exercise to be applied for effective results. It is a good choice to exercise, even when you may not be working on maintaining a weight goal. Exercise can also lift up your mood. If you choose a dance routine, it can put you in a happy mind-frame. Remember, that walking, running and stretching, is always good for the muscles to keep you mobile.

Some resent studies are stating that we may not need to exercise to lose weight. One of the reasons why exercise is a form of weight loss is that it helps us to burn off fat. Losing weight means just that. Fat has to be lost (excreted), from our bodies. When we exercise we sweat and fat is burned off.

If you have a diet plan and you are not excreting off fat, your weight loss can be slow or non-effective. Some simple ways to cleanse off fat are drinking tea daily, eating more salads, adding probiotics to your meals, drinking warm lemon water, before food in the morning. You can also have prune juice with your dinner, or eat a few prunes before bed time.

Fibers are needed to clear fat in stool. Being regular daily is not sufficient to lose weight and burn off fat. Fat must be excreted from our bodies to reduce bloating in our stomach and weight retention. Always work with what is right for you.

Movement keeps us mobile, burns fat and gives energy.

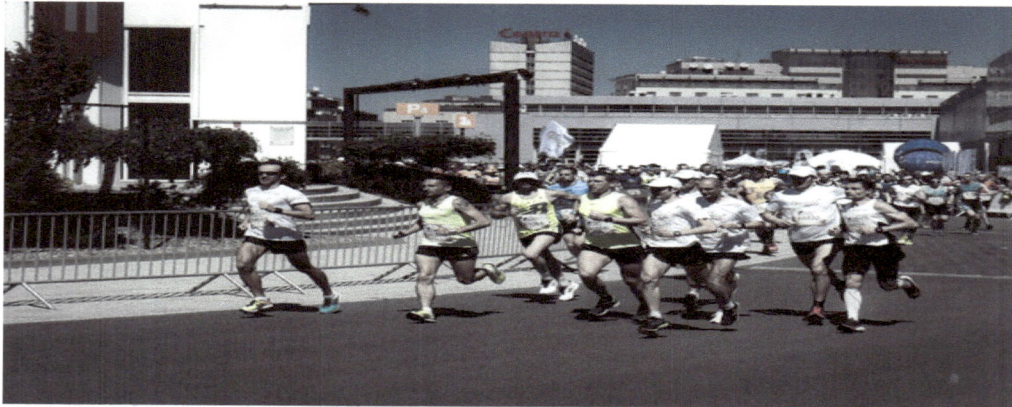

Five

Attraction

Have you ever heard of the word, "Attraction?" The Universal Law of Attraction, that is. Now you are probably asking about now...
"What in the world does attraction have to do with my diet plan?"

May I ask you a personal question? You are reading this alone, I gather, so answering this question is private, yes? Just between us. Have you ever been attracted to some one in your life? Your answer... "Aw... yes! But?

Well did you fall for that person whom you were attracted to? Don't want to admit it. Most likely you were drown to them yes? You were drawn in as they say, "Like a moth to a flame."

Your answer, "Yeah ... Kinda, well, yes.

Here is the thing, this is a simple way to explain the Law of Attraction. I am sorry if anyone have told you before now,   that you should just believe that it works. You see knowledge is power, therefore you need to know and understand what you are learning and doing, in order to apply it correctly, or efficiently.

Attraction causes us to take notice and be drawn in by our senses. Our five senses cause what we call, "Like attracts like." Think about that for a second. If you like the way a person smell, you are most likely to be drawn to them, yes? If you do not like a fragrance, it can repel you, yes?

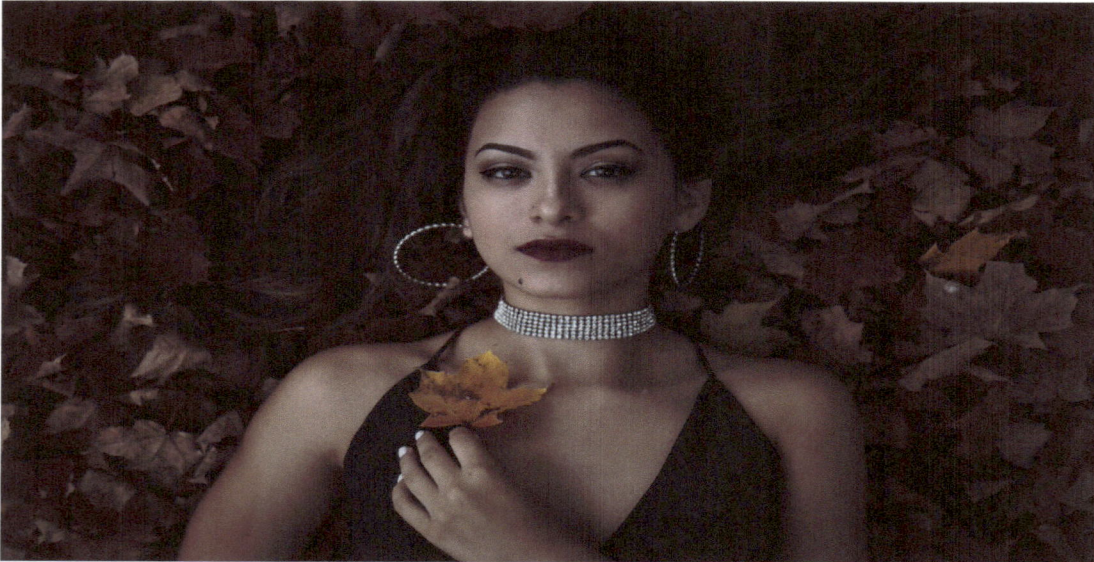

Now here is the kicker. When it comes to diet, most of us really like food. We like the taste of it, its smell, the different textures of food, the sizzling sound of the fryer and the picture perfect displays that confronts us. These senses are all natural and they tells us that we can have food. We can be nourished and satisfied. They are signals to our brain, to sustain and preserve our life.

When ever we are attracted to something, it happens because it is something that we want. Our senses then picks up on that corresponding side of desire, like the joining of two magnets which are negative and positive, to make a positive whole.

Attraction is real. The Law of Attraction is real. It works whether you are aware of it or not. It works whether you think that what you experience maybe only coincidences. You are desiring food and it is coming to you. Yes, this law works for everything, even food.

When you have a plan and you are working on it, it will work for you. However, the food that you desire is also coming to you by attraction, each and every time you think of it. If you ate every two hours, you will be always thinking about what to eat next.

Food will be foremost on your mind, and therefore you will be attraction more of it. You will be constantly looking for what you have available to enjoy to eat. It is all about the food for you, while you may believe that it is the diet. In this understanding, you can see that it is not the diet, but the food being the focus point.

Attraction = Like Attracts Like

So how do you manage this challenge? Continue on to the next chapter to **discover your answer.**

Eat Healthy and Live Well

Fruits and vegetables are composed of necessary nutrients, which we need in our diet. Are you always attracting the right amounts for your daily needs?

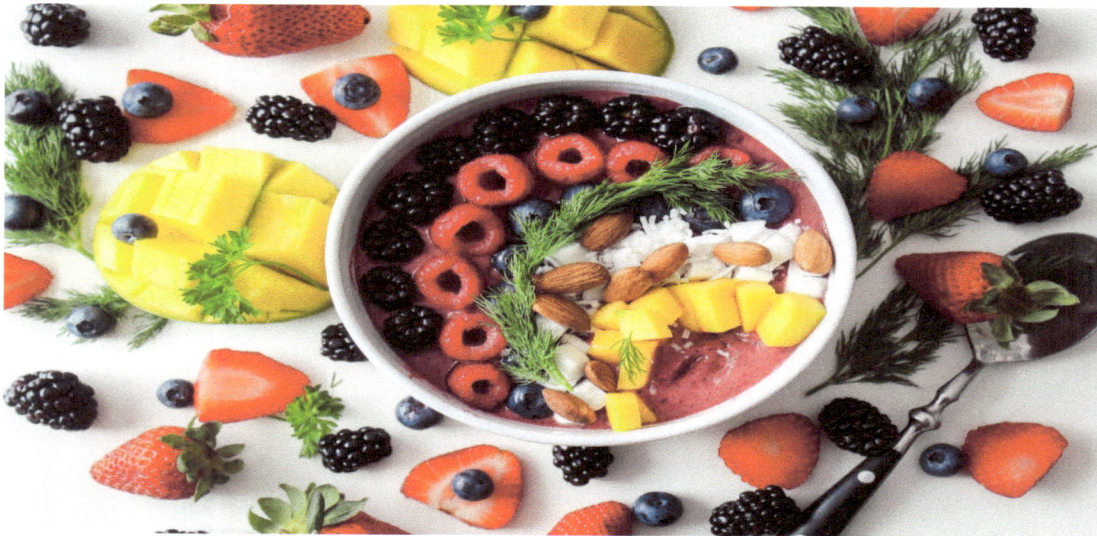

Six

Balancing Life

The phrase, "Balancing life", can mean different things to different people. What exactly does it mean for you? Do you think of juggling several things at once? Look at your life. Is there enough time in your day to accomplish all the activities that you will like to achieve? Or, can you set aside the needed time?

Does your day revolve around work, chores, children, spouse and family? Not to mention that you may also have sports, church activities and board memberships meetings, to attend. It can be a lot to manage on a daily basis.

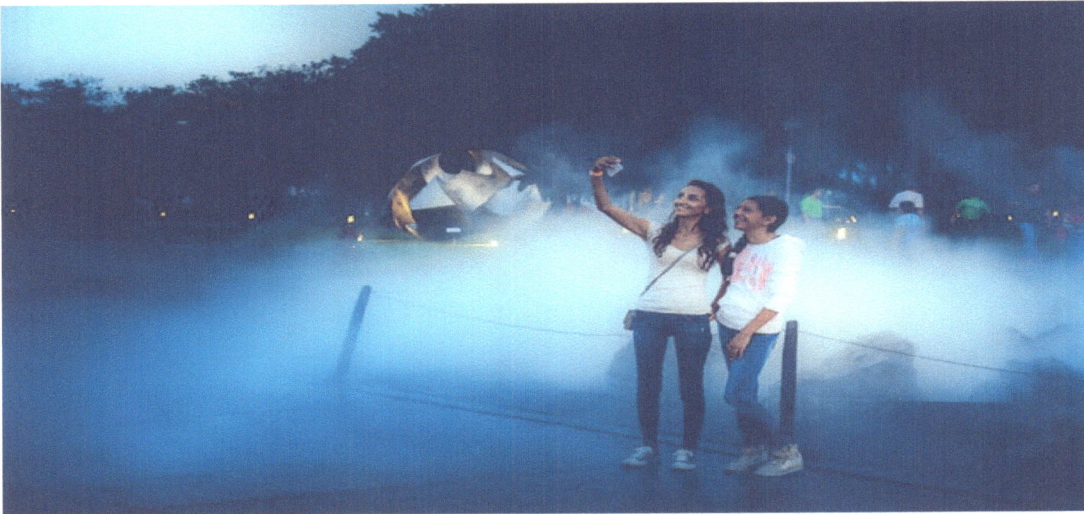

Balancing Life

Do you have a balance life? Do you think that a balance life is even necessary? When ever you look around in our society today your answer to me may be, "Everyone is doing it..." Everyone is to busy to be bothered with being balanced. Who has the time to plan such goals, far more to be able to achieve them.

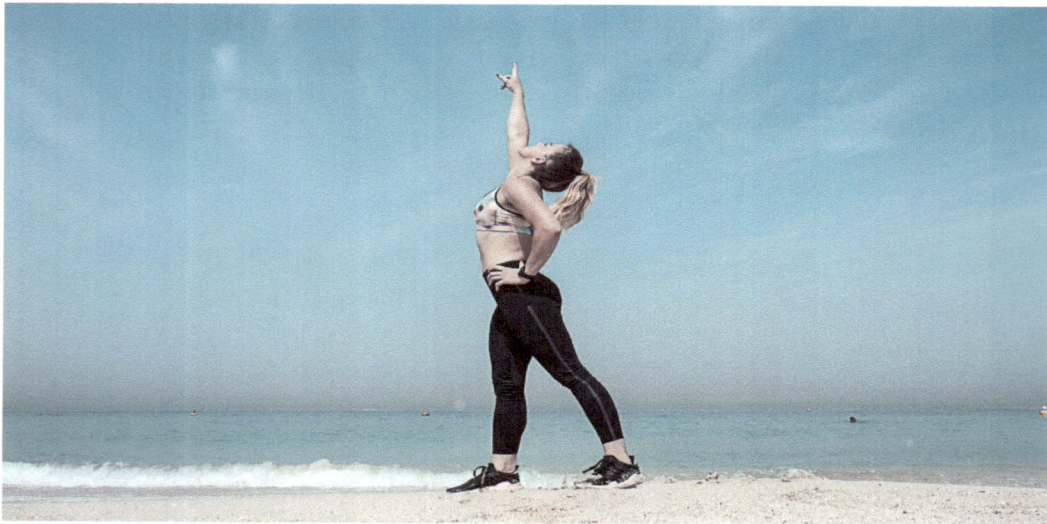

The truth is, while we are young and healthy balance is not considered by many as important. The twenties and thirties age group seldom goes to the doctor for annual check ups. It is only when they have a sudden ailment, that the doctor is considered. The statistics on this are proven.

In the age of maturity however, we become more thoughtful of yearly checks and balancing our lives. Our bodies reminds us that we need to care for it. We may look back and hold different views of what we could have done differently. Those choices includes health, relationships, career and money, in sometimes that order. One of the importance of balancing our lives you see does affect our health.

Aging affects our choices not only to eat healthy and exercise, but it help us to work on our stress levels. Stress is one of the key factors in eating and health issues for us today. Stress can cause us to make choices, which we may not have made without it. Balancing our life can help our stress levels and our health, including our need for dieting.

Let us look at what stress can actually do to our diet plans.

When you work with a trainer you may have a lot of benefits. However, don't get into the idea that this is the only thing to do. You can have the wrong understanding and habits which the brain accepts to please. Falling from one habit to the other, is not always right, and will not change your desired outcome.

A trainer can work with you, either on your exercise goals, or with your diet goals. After your trainers are gone, the habits which you have developed, are what you will need to keep you focus and on track.

Your Target

If you will like to lose weight and keep it off, you must also have a permanent target. For example, you may choose to lose 10 pounds to fit into a dress or clothing for a special occasion. That target can easily be reached. However, once you have obtained that target, there is no more **why,** you should maintain the new weight. Your focus can be lost and your old weight regained.

You need a great "**Why,**" to do anything. For maintaining your weight, **the secret is "Lifestyle."** . Why? It is a lifestyle to live in a height that will help you to feel comfortable and healthy. To look and feel better. No more rubbing legs, tiredness and ill fitting clothes. When you lose fifty pounds, or enough weight to have that comfort, it will be easier for you to say no to foods and portions, that does not support the new you.

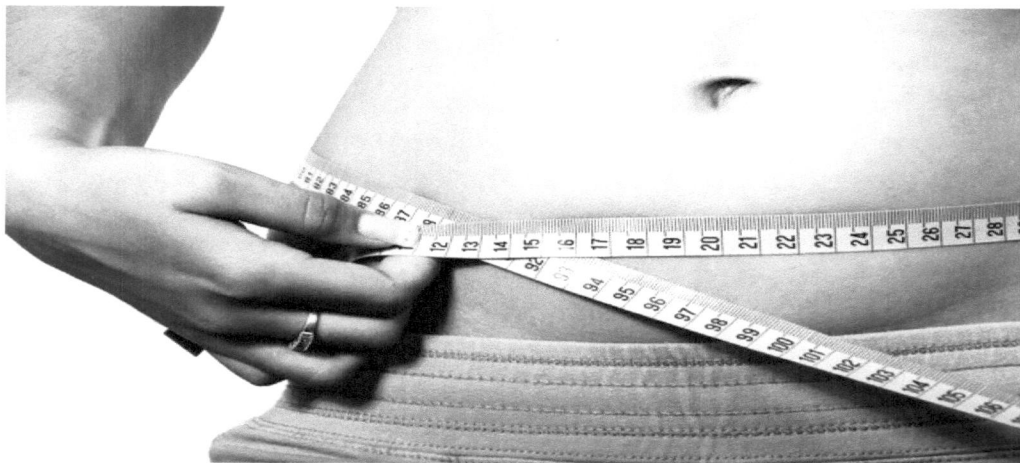

Seven

Self Rewards

Here is a little trouble waiting to happen.

Do you have or ever had a dog? Do you know of anyone who has a dog? Have you ever seen how some dog owners train their dog? They say a command, example.."Sit." The dog then sits and next a treat is given for compliance to the command.

After sometime, the dog will sit without the command if he sees you holding the treat. This is how we train the brain. It is easier when we expect a reward. We get that good feeling. Self rewards helps us feel deserving. Similar like the dog that sits for the treat.

I do hope that I am not offending you by using this analogy. It is the simplest way that I can help you to see, how training the brain with expectation works. Some people do this with their children. They offer rewards such as, going to the park, game or movies, for cleaning their room and completing home chores.

You know, of cause, the littered room full of clothes and books becomes clean in under and hour. You know what I am talking about, yes? You may have done it too, as a child, or received rewards for doing so. Rewards are a common practice.

We are trained in rewards for food, pasting test and doing chores. Don't get me wrong. You should celebrate your achievements but whenever we are rewarded with food, to break a diet, it is a chance to form a pattern, which the brain can come to expect.

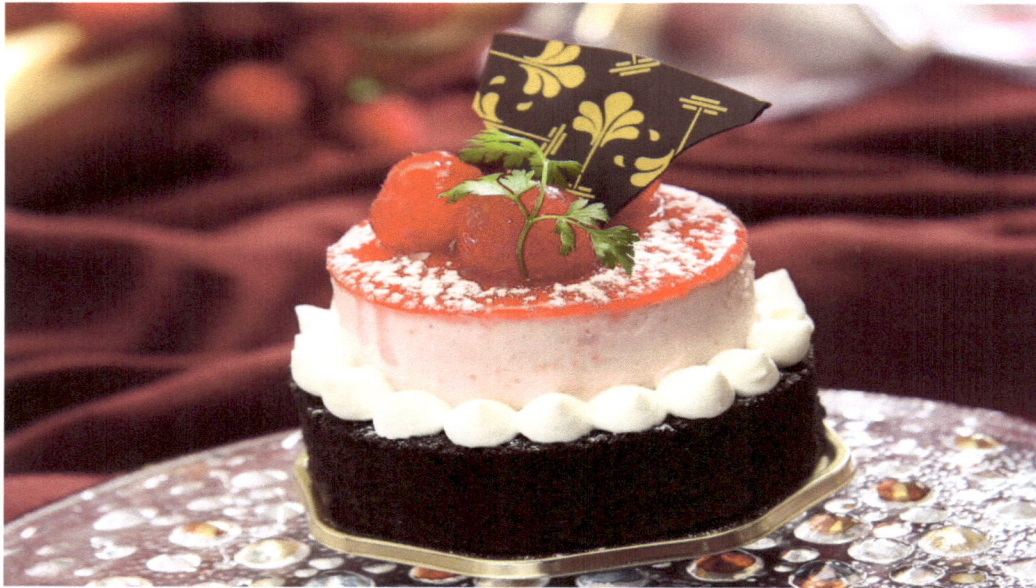

Keeping a diet plan, may then be harder to accomplish. If anyone tells you that its okay, go ahead and have that little snack reward, be careful. Be sure that it is something that you can have control over. Otherwise it can form guilt and lead to a larger challenge. You should not expect it to be okay, to break away from your plan without any effects on (not only) you gaining weight but taking your focus off course.

Keep your rewards to a minimum. Remember that you are already doing something, which you chose to be right for you. There is no need for further rewards, but to write in your journal and feel the self satisfaction of your accomplishment. Know that you are doing so well. Be pleased with yourself.

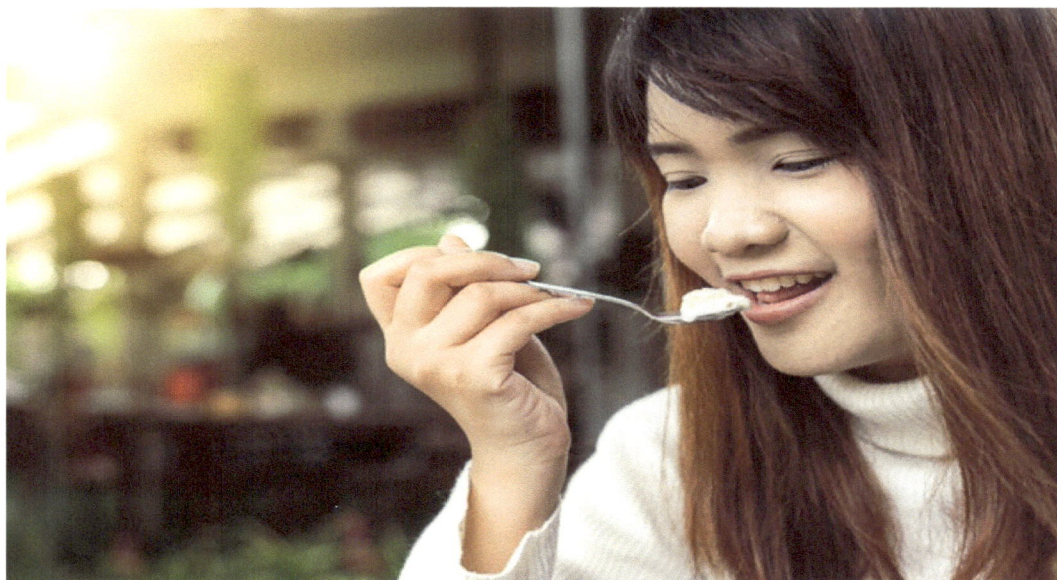

When you celebrate you can also have smaller portions. Remember that sometimes just a little can be enjoyed to go a long way in fulfillment.

Next is what you can do, to achieve maintenance of your diet goals.

Eight

Personal Development

Taking you to your next level, personal development will help you to learn more about yourself, your mindset, beliefs and where they were formed, for you.

It is like learning about your ancestry, where they came from. Personal development can help you to better understand your health challenges, by understanding your beliefs. You can gain new awareness, which will allow you to make different choices.

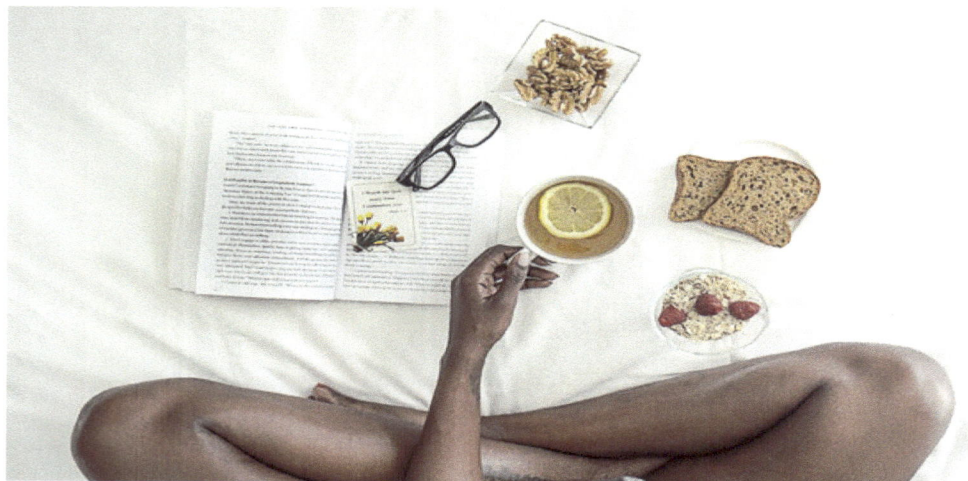

Finding the cause and changing them to new habits that works, with personal development.

The way by which we do thing comes largely from our nature and nurture. When we are aware of ourselves, our comfort zone (that we need to come out of it), only then can change be accomplished. You can learn (by this means), how to balance your stress, health and life.

Through personal development you can learn how most of your challenges begins with fear. Fear is a balance in our emotions that can help us to be careful of danger. However, we give it far to much authority in our lives. We are not taught how fear works, why it works and how we can override it.

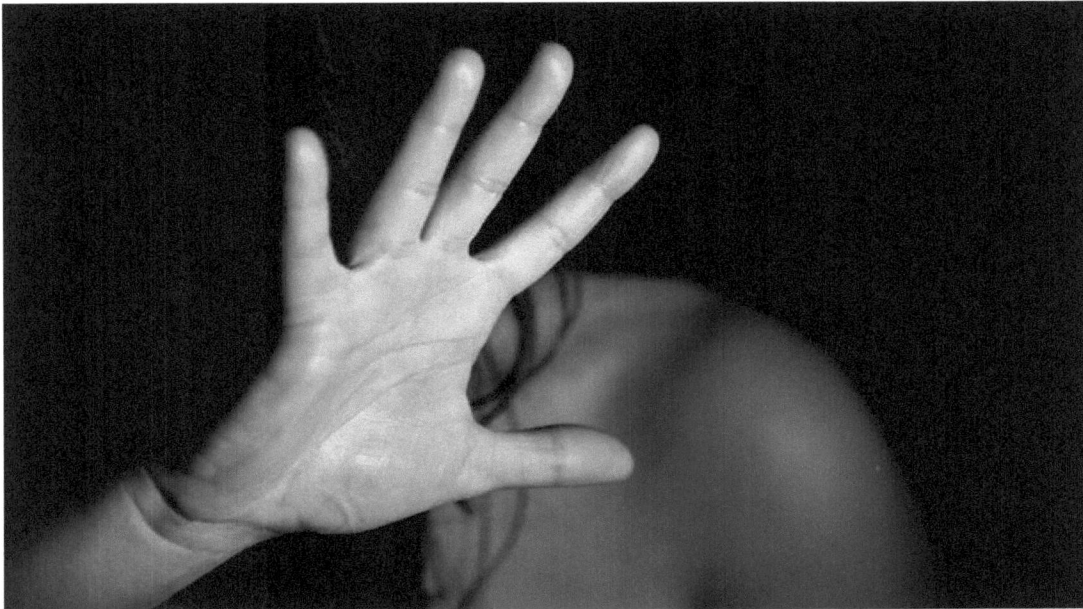

Since most of our beliefs are formed from our childhood and as young adults, with a developing brain not yet matured, (the mind matures at 25-26 years, in decision making abilities), we can begin to see our fears came from a lack of knowledge and information, viewed by a child's mind.

That lack of knowledge and information is why we fear. Now here is how we fear. Our emotions carry the memory of experience of fear to our brain, based on lack of information. Those experiences which were attained in our nurture and environment, can be a cause of how we fear.

Maturity by itself does not teach us how to overcome any past memories. It can cause us to further hold on to those memories, as part of our life experiences. Gaining information by way of reading and research, can help us to dive further into our past, to uncover our feeling of fear and of our beliefs. It can allow us a path to change, once the discovery is made.

The brain stores all things which we see, hear, smell, touch and taste, but also how we feel emotionally. Changing the recorded memory (which were formed while we were still immature and developing in judgment), we can change the story in our brain.

This is called, "Brain training". We are already trained by our emotions (like our rewards to feel good), so retraining our brain is now necessary. It is like a computer, where you need to delete unwanted data and replace it with new up-to-date information, that is relative for your usage.

Some of the training that helps our brain are by using positive affirmations, vision boards, visualization and subliminal messages. These methods are used to retrain our brain, on the subconscious level.

Retraining your brain to serve your new interest with understanding, is the maximum benefit for you. You will find the consistency which you require, when you build new beliefs and habits, which will support your plan.

These affirmations can also be used on your vision board. Read them daily, to stay on track and keep your focus.

Mind Training Affirmations

I am in the best of health.
I live a healthy lifestyle daily.
Food nourishes my body to health.
My body only takes what it needs to be nourished.
Rest gives me a clear mindset.
I am rejuvenated by food and sleep.
I eat what I chose to be nourished.
I love my personal growth and development.

Nine

The Secret's Out

Since you have completed the previous chapters, you should have a better understanding, that it takes more than a diet plan, to maintain a diet goal.

We have talked about how the brain works to form habits. You are enlightened about the human desire and attraction for food. You came to see that we live in the practice of rewards for our behaviors. You have learned that, by the you practicing personal development, you can retrain your brain, to make different choices based on new information and knowledge, and so attaining your goal.

In brain training you can begin with a vision board. You can make a board with pictures and affirmations to keep you focus and on track to your goal. These pictures works well for people who are visual learners. The next will be visualization. This technique or method, allows you to form a mental picture of you, in the way that you will like to be and live.

Next, meditation can help with stress to keep you calm. It works by you breathing deeply and sending enough oxygen to your brain. The last method of using subliminal recordings, will train the brain further, when combined with the previous methods. In the practicing of these methods you are personalizing what works for you. Not a one size fit all lifestyle.

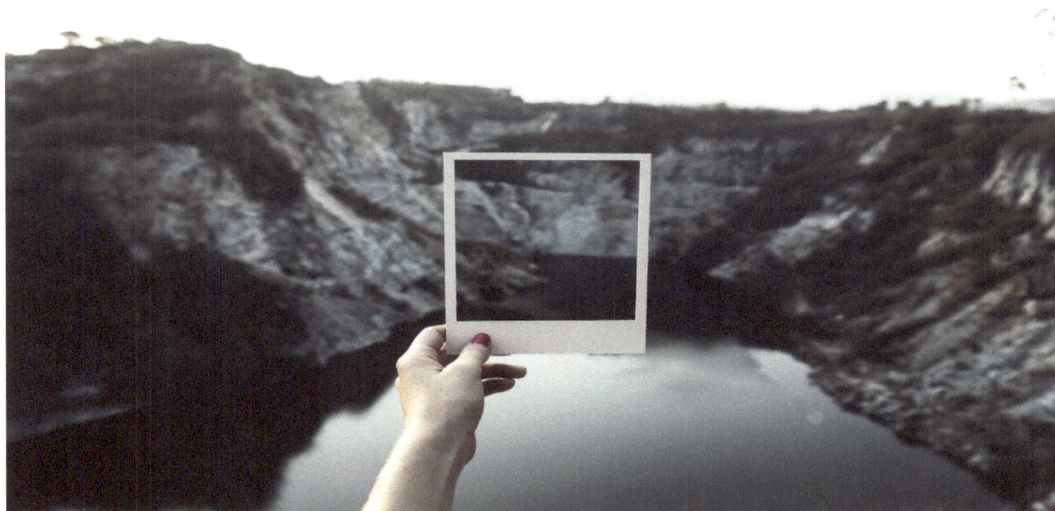

When you add self-control, self-confidence and self- awareness in your new understanding, you can begin to be the conqueror, of your habits. Yes, I said conqueror, because not having to live for food, but by food is a part of conquering a habit.

We need more than food to live a healthy, stress free life. We need self-love. The kind of love that preserves us. The kind that cares for us. The desire to be our best that we can possible be. Make your weight one of which you are comfortable in your own skin. Your looks tell of your confidence and choice. Your health speaks of your energy and alertness. This is you. No one else. And, you have it all.

This is Your Secret.

It takes Courage

What is courage and what does it take to have courage for you? Courage is doing something even when there is fear of doing it and we are unsure of the outcome. Courage is knowing what we cannot change, what we can change and understanding the difference, to apply it to our choices. When we apply courage, it gave us strength to follow through with our plans.

You Have the key Ingredients

It takes Strength

It takes strength to change. Especially if you are facing a challenge alone. Courage needs to be applied to first look into the situation, and then be honest with your findings. Secondly, to then act on them so that you can create the change that you want.

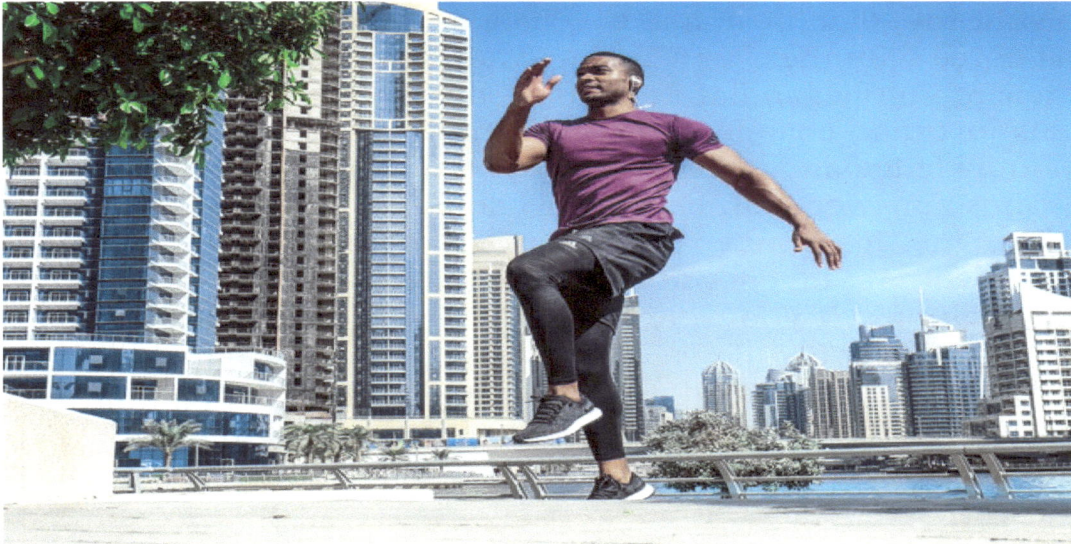

Find the strength by holding on to your "why," you want or need, this change in your life. Strength is simple letting go of some fears, while being aware that the fears are there. You are a conqueror. You have the courage and strength. Again you can find support to carry you through your plan, with your efforts. A forum can be a good place to start.

Ten

New Habits

Knowledge is power, only when it is applied. Everything you have read in this book, whether you agree with it or not, will not make a change for you by itself. It is only if you apply this new knowledge to your life, that it can make a change for you.

If you don't agree with these new understanding, or apply them, you can stay where you began before reading this book. To make a change means just that, change. You must find what to change, and what new knowledge and understanding you will need to make your change. Those answers can help your choice, which will aid your desired outcome. Remember that, change can not follow the right direction for you, if you choose the wrong direction.

Look at this example. If you were following directions to get to a destination and you went down the wrong street, you may become lost. However, if you had a map, (or GPS) and was able to find a connecting street to where you had intended to go, only then you can find your way to your desired destination.

Your Alignment For the Next Level

What is this alignment? You maybe asking. Why do I need it? Well here is the thing that most of us is not aware of. Alignment is getting two sides of something to work together or have and exact fit. It is having that matching part or for this analogy, finding your connected street.

Here is why you need alignment. There can be some reason why your mind maybe set on a diet, which can cause you to always feel hungry. One reason can be, because you are out of alignment. This is sometimes called, "A medical condition".

Working on only a diet at this stage, could be like trying to cut an object with a small knife, which is two feet away form you. When you are able to bring the object within your reach, only then, that the cutting action can be carried out effectively.

It is quite obvious that you cannot maintain a diet if you are always hungry. This is only one kind of challenge. What ever your challenge may be, you must first recognize and understand it. Then with help you can begin to work on bringing them into alignment, to get your diet plan working for you.

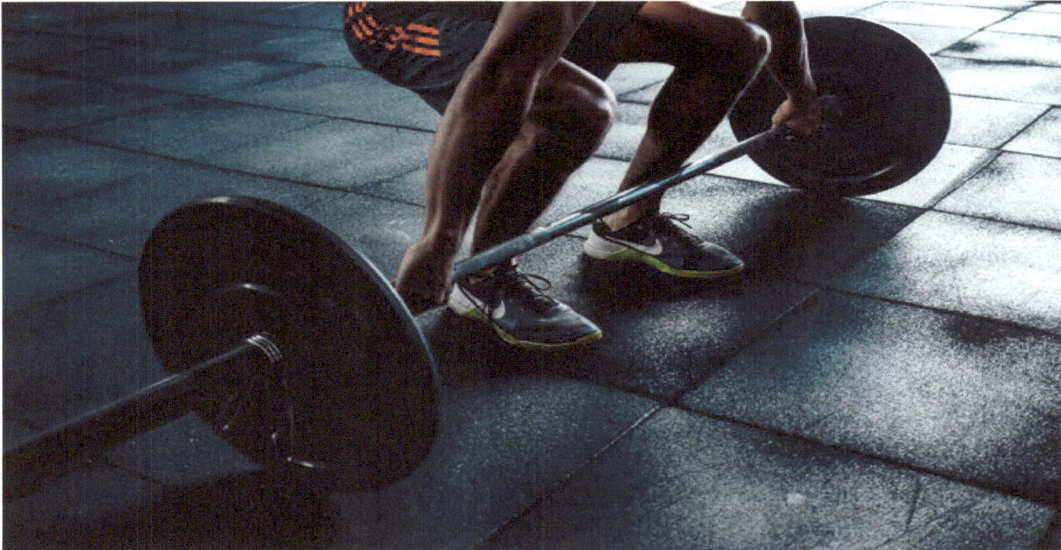

Making changes and developing new habits, allows us to go to the next level of development. Forming new beliefs about who we are and what we can accomplish, is one of the foundations for growth.

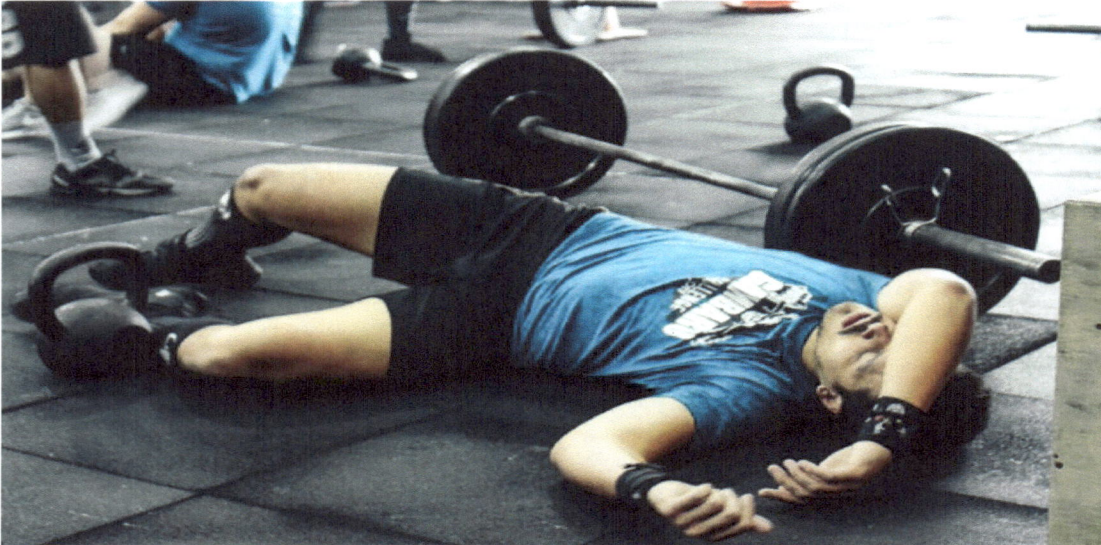

You may have asked why others have used a diet plan and it has worked for them. The truth is that some people can stick to a plan for different reasons, while others can not. Not everyone finds it easy to follow a routine without help. Help may be needed to follow a plan, based on your beliefs and life habits, which has become normal for you.

Whether a coach on personal development or health, using help can be the aid, that you need to change. They can guide you to make better choices, for you to achieve your goals.

Work on treating the cause of your dietary issues or condition and not just the effects of them. Most conditions carry causes and effects, which is another universal Law. Example, choosing an unhealthy choice can cause ill health. The understanding once again, is how to work within the Universal Laws, which can be studied and applied, through personal growth and development.

We have already discussed the Law of Attraction, where you saw how like attracts like. Thinking about what you want and making it the best for you, will in fact attract just that. You will begin to see all around you, things which are good for you, showing up for you. They will all come in naturally for you, as you become aware of them.

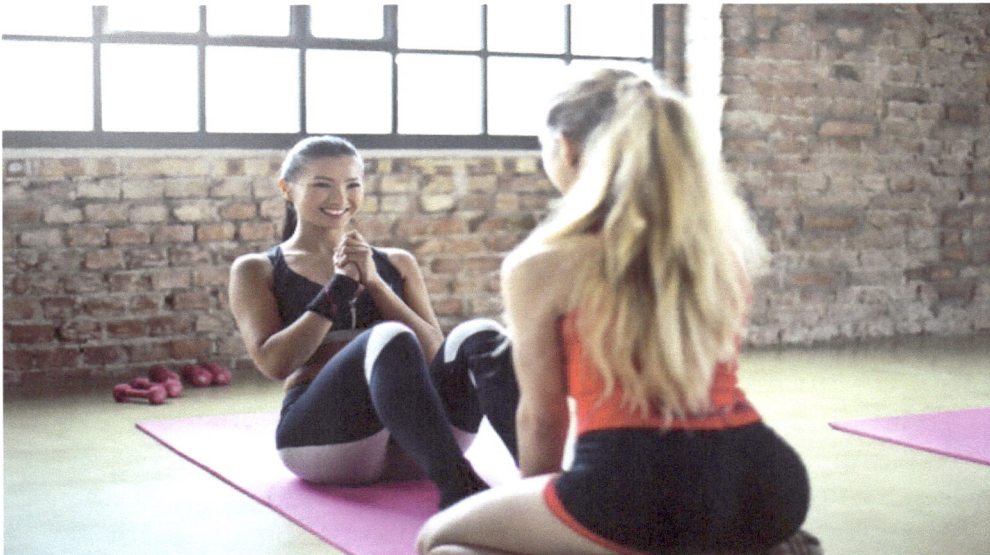

Here are some healthy choices which you can add to your new diet lifestyle.

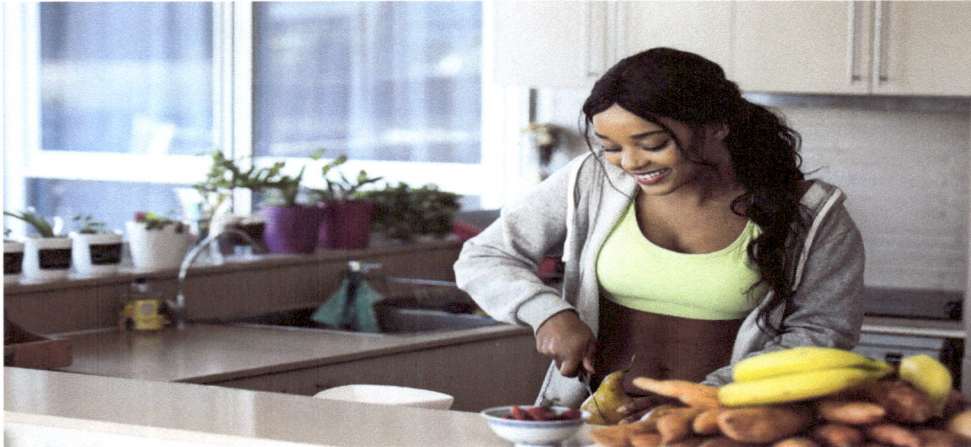

When you work with maintaining fruits and vegetables in your diet plan, some super healthy foods are avocado and beet. Beets are anti-inflammatory, high in fibers, detoxing and has a verity of nutritional benefits for your diet. While avocado has nutritional benefits for the liver, kidney, eyes, and blood pressure, as does beets. You can research to learn more about these great vegetables.

Here is one of my personal favorites and simple recipe, which my mother made for me as a child, so that I would eat beets. You can use your potato salad recipe and add beets to it. Your children may just love it too, if you prepare it for them on the holidays. You can also add the beet juice to your green tea. When you steam your beets, use the water to add to your tea. Use this only for fresh beets from your supermarket, not if you are using can or jar beets. (which are already sliced). Can and jar beets, can only be used for the salad.

If you are using fresh beets, you can try saving a ½ cup or so, of the red water and store it in a tightly covered bottle, then place in your refrigerator. When you are ready to make your tea, you can add a ¼ of a cup to your tea, with a bit of honey. This will add more fiber and antioxidant to your nutritional intake at tea time.

Enjoy Your Red Tea. It is Delicious!

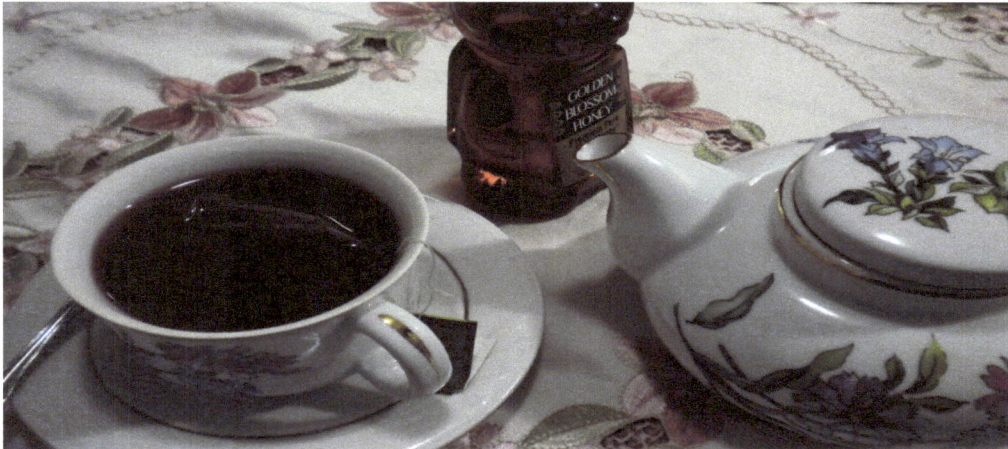

Photo of my personal tea time.

Beets are also good in salads and soups. You can research some recipes and try them out, to find out which one of them, that you enjoy the best. But, whether cold or hot, adding this food to your meal plan, will offer you much nutritional benefits.

Recipe for Beet Salad

Ingredients:

1 Medium Beet
2 Large Potatoes
1 Celery Stalk
¼ Slice Small Onion
1 Medium Carrot
Salt and Ground White Pepper
2 Tbsp Mayonnaise

Wash and steam vegetables until they are tender when pierced. Cook beets for about 15 minutes. **Don't over cook** to loose the nutritional value. Potatoes may take a bit longer. Chop vegetables (once cooled), into cubes for salad. Add salt and pepper to taste, (about a pinch). Combine all ingredients to make a pretty pink salad. Served chilled. Decorate with celery leaves.

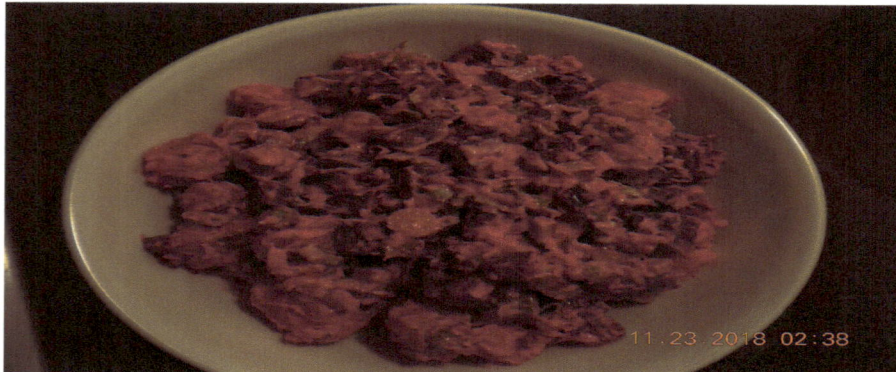

Photo of my homemade salad recipe.

Seeking a life coach, along with your dietary plan is, "The Secret," to you achieving your goal. Don't just think you can diet. Get to the root cause of your challenge. Work to get the maximum results from the diet plan you are working with.

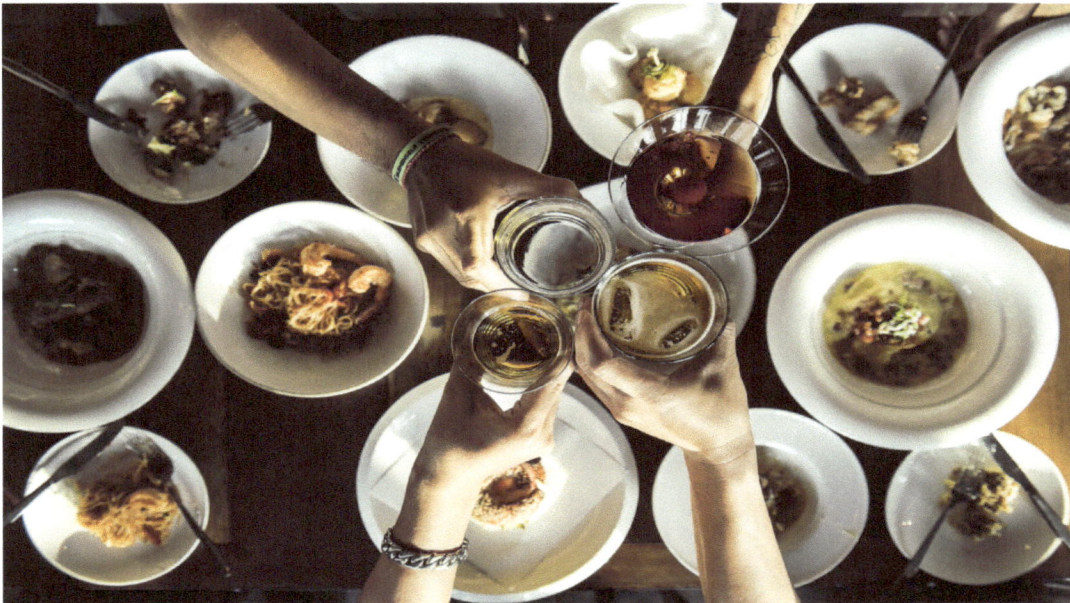

You can overcome your weight or health condition, to be your ideal self. You are much stronger than you may think. Do some research and apply what you have learn. Study your options, but don't get bugged down. Don't over think your answer, seek help and do it. Taking the first right action, is what can bring you greater results.

My New Habits

You will be on a path to self-confidence. This is your body, your health and your life choices. When you are able to get to this stage, you will no longer feel the frustration of yo yo dieting (the struggle to say **no,** to over eating) and other choices that may be challenging for you.

Make your diet goal one of a new lifestyle habit. Add personal development. Become aware of your choices. Find the cause of your challenges. Grow into the new you and live the life that you were meant to live. **Be the best you, that you can be!**

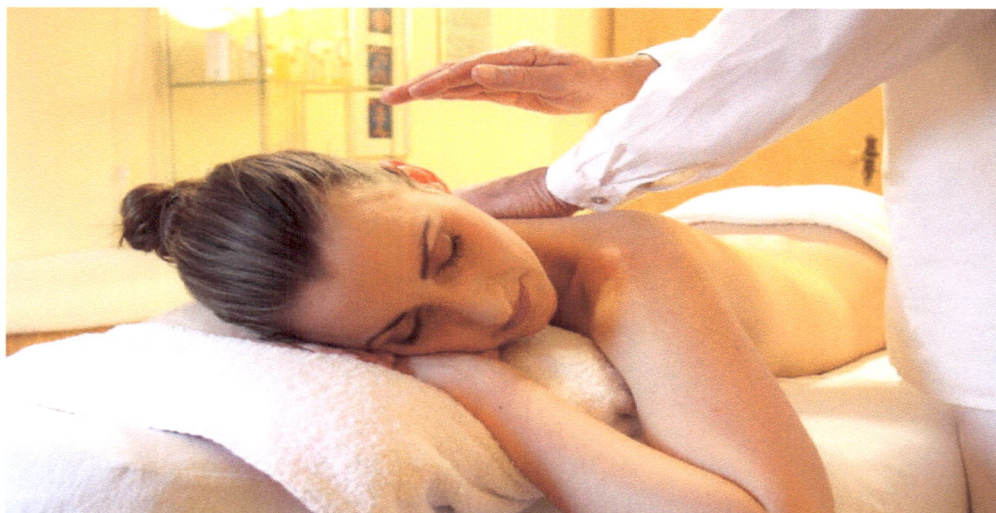

Enjoy Your Journey. Live Well!

Conclusion

You may have picked up this book to read, with the thought that there is no secret to diet. You simple eat what you like.

In the interim, for some people who have been struggling with weight loss or over eating, the idea that they may be missing something, is quite possible. They may in fact imagine, that there can be, "A Secret to Diet."

Well, finally the secret is out. You now hold the secret. You can use it, or pass it on and share it. You now hold the missing piece, in the puzzle of your diet.

Sorry if you were expecting rocket science. This is not it. That you can research for yourself. Science is also being shared as they come available, in today's media. However, most solutions are really much larger or simpler, than we see them.

Finding someone to tell you the secret to diet is found here in this book. It is more than your diet. Personal development, your mind and lifestyle, is the change that you need to see more, think deeper and to believe in yourself. I know you can do this.

Live well, learn all that you can and be awesome!

About the Author

I am JJ Schousboe, a certified Life Coach by the Global Science Foundation and the Center of Personal Reinvention as a Relationships Coach. A lifetime member of Strathmore's WHO'S WHO, I was awarded Strathmore's WHO'S WHO Worldwide, Woman of Excellence. I am also the president of JJ Learning Curve, LLC, a wife, mother and lives in Florida, USA.

I have written a series of personal development course books, to help those who are aspiring to get to the next level of self help and achievement.

An educator for some twenty years, it is my dearest desire to share my knowledge to help and inspire others by my company's motto:

To An Amplified Life. Bridging the gap from academics to your life's achievement.

You can learn more about me and my services at: **http://jjlearningcurve.com**

Resources

JJ Learning Curve, LLC
http://jjlearningcurve.com

Book Store

https://lulu.com/spotlight/Joanne18
https://www.jjlearningcurve.com/shop

MASTERING IT!

Three Course Series
Mastering It... Learn To Love
Relationships Development –
Series One

Mastering It... Envision You
Visualization Development –
Series Two

Mastering It... Crown Your Achievements
Spiritual and Personal Development –
Series Three

Awakening to Words of Wisdom

www.ingramcontent.com/pod-product-compliance
Lightning Source LLC
Chambersburg PA
CBHW060809270326
41928CB00002B/39